FROM TRAUMA TO TRIUMPH:
The Mental Resilience of Brazilian Jiu-Jitsu

How to Build Good Habits and Break Bad Ones

By

JOAO CRUS

Table of Contents

CHAPTER 1

Understanding Trauma and Its Impact

Defining Trauma

Trauma can be a complex and multifaceted experience that affects individuals on various levels. It is often defined as a deeply distressing or disturbing experience that leaves a lasting impact on a person's mental, emotional, and physical well-being. This can include events such as physical or emotional abuse, accidents, the loss of a loved one, or any situation that overwhelms an individual's ability to cope. Understanding trauma in a broader context helps to recognize its diverse manifestations, from anxiety and depression to issues with self-esteem and interpersonal relationships.

The effects of trauma are not solely psychological; they can also manifest physically. Individuals may experience chronic pain, fatigue, or other somatic symptoms as a result of their trauma. In many cases, these physical symptoms can complicate the healing process, making it difficult for individuals to engage in activities that promote well-being, such as exercise. This is particularly relevant for adults who may be overweight or sedentary, as they may find it challenging to participate in physical activities like Brazilian Jiu-Jitsu (BJJ) that could facilitate healing and personal growth.

BJJ offers a unique approach to overcoming trauma by emphasizing physical movement and the development of mental resilience. The practice involves grappling techniques that require focus, discipline, and a sense of control, all of which can be beneficial for those dealing with the aftermath of traumatic experiences. Engaging in BJJ not only encourages physical fitness but also fosters an environment where individuals can build confidence and self-esteem. As practitioners learn to navigate challenging situations on the mat, they can begin to draw parallels to their personal struggles, enabling them to confront and process their trauma in a supportive space.

The integration of emotional intelligence into BJJ coaching can enhance the therapeutic benefits of the practice. Coaches who understand the psychological aspects of trauma can create tailored experiences that cater to the emotional needs of their students. This can include teaching mindfulness techniques, promoting positive self-talk, and encouraging open discussions about mental health. By fostering a culture of awareness and support, BJJ academies can become safe havens for individuals seeking to overcome their pasts and build a brighter future.

Lastly, BJJ serves as a powerful tool for personal growth and goal setting, particularly for women who may face unique challenges related to empowerment and emotional regulation. The sport encourages participants to step out of their comfort zones, confront fears, and develop a sense of agency over their bodies and lives. As individuals progress in their training, they not only improve their physical capabilities but also cultivate resilience, emotional strength, and a renewed sense of purpose. In this way, BJJ transcends its role as a martial art and emerges as a transformative practice that fosters healing and growth in the face of trauma.

The Psychological Effects of Trauma

Trauma can have profound and lasting psychological effects that influence an individual's emotional and mental well-being. Many adults, particularly those who have experienced significant life challenges, may find themselves grappling with anxiety, depression, and low self-esteem. These psychological burdens often manifest as physical symptoms, disrupting daily life and inhibiting personal growth. Understanding the psychological effects of trauma is crucial for those seeking pathways to recovery and resilience, especially within the context of Brazilian Jiu-Jitsu (BJJ), which serves as both a physical and mental training ground.

The impact of trauma can lead to feelings of disconnection, overwhelming stress, and a heightened state of anxiety. For individuals struggling with sedentary lifestyles or those who feel overwhelmed by their circumstances, the idea of engaging in physical activities can seem daunting. However, BJJ provides an environment where individuals can gradually confront their fears and anxieties. The practice encourages participants to step outside their comfort zones, which can be a powerful catalyst for emotional healing. By learning to navigate physical challenges on the mat, practitioners often find parallels in their ability to manage emotional challenges off the mat.

Building confidence and self-esteem is essential for overcoming the psychological effects of trauma. Brazilian Jiu-Jitsu emphasizes personal growth through progressive skill development, which can help individuals recognize their strengths. As practitioners learn new techniques and achieve small victories, they cultivate a sense of accomplishment that fosters self-worth. This journey can lead to significant shifts in how individuals perceive themselves, enabling them to break free from the limiting beliefs often instilled by past traumas. In this way, BJJ becomes not only a sport but a transformative experience that instills resilience and self-assurance.

Emotional intelligence plays a vital role in both coaching and practice within the BJJ community. Coaches who integrate emotional intelligence into their teaching methods can create a supportive environment that acknowledges the psychological barriers their students may face. By fostering open communication and encouraging vulnerability, coaches can help practitioners develop skills in emotional regulation. This not only enhances their performance on the mat but also equips them with tools to manage their emotions in everyday life. The supportive nature of the BJJ community further contributes to this growth, allowing individuals to feel connected and understood.

Ultimately, Brazilian Jiu-Jitsu serves as a powerful tool for personal growth and goal setting. For many, engaging in BJJ represents a commitment to self-improvement that encompasses both physical and mental dimensions. As practitioners set and achieve goals, whether related to technique, fitness, or competition, they build a sense of purpose and direction. This process of goal achievement can be particularly empowering for women, who may face unique challenges related to trauma and self-regulation. By fostering an inclusive and empowering environment, BJJ can help individuals reclaim their narratives, transforming trauma into triumph and fostering a lifelong journey of resilience and strength.

The Importance of Mental Resilience

Mental resilience is a critical attribute that enables individuals to navigate life's challenges, particularly in the face of adversity. In the context of Brazilian Jiu-Jitsu (BJJ), mental resilience plays a pivotal role not only in the physical aspects of the sport but also in fostering emotional strength. For adults, whether they are new to the practice, professionals, or individuals seeking a healthier lifestyle, developing mental resilience through BJJ can lead to significant improvements in overall well-being. This process involves cultivating a mindset that embraces challenges, learns from setbacks, and remains steadfast in the pursuit of personal goals.

BJJ provides an effective platform for building confidence and self-esteem. As practitioners grapple with opponents and learn complex techniques, they are often forced to confront their fears and insecurities. This engagement in physical struggle fosters an environment where individuals can push beyond their perceived limits. Each small victory on the mat, whether it's successfully executing a technique or overcoming a more experienced opponent, contributes to a growing sense of self-efficacy. This self-assurance, cultivated through rigorous training and practice, translates into everyday life, enabling individuals to tackle personal and professional challenges with greater confidence.

Emotional intelligence is another crucial component of mental resilience, and BJJ inherently emphasizes this aspect. Through the interactions with coaches and training partners, practitioners learn to read social cues, manage their emotions, and respond to stress in a constructive manner. Coaches who integrate emotional intelligence into their teaching approach can help students recognize their emotional responses during training and competition. This awareness not only enhances performance on the mat but also equips individuals with strategies to manage anxiety and stress in their daily lives, effectively improving their mental resilience.

For many, the journey through trauma can feel isolating and overwhelming. However, BJJ offers a supportive community that fosters healing and personal growth. The act of rolling on the mat requires vulnerability and trust, both of which are essential for overcoming past traumas. As individuals learn to face physical challenges, they simultaneously confront emotional obstacles. The discipline and mental toughness developed through BJJ create a pathway to recovery, helping practitioners replace feelings of helplessness with empowerment and agency in their own lives.

Furthermore, BJJ serves as a powerful tool for personal growth and goal setting. The structured nature of the sport encourages practitioners to set objectives, whether it be mastering a particular technique or preparing for a competition. This goal-oriented mindset reinforces the principles of perseverance and hard work, essential elements of mental resilience. Female empowerment is particularly evident in BJJ, where women are increasingly taking up the sport and finding strength in their physicality and mental fortitude. The inclusive nature of BJJ allows individuals from all backgrounds to experience emotional regulation and personal empowerment, ultimately fostering a community that champions resilience and growth.

CHAPTER 2

Introduction to Brazilian Jiu-Jitsu

The History of Brazilian Jiu-Jitsu

Brazilian Jiu-Jitsu (BJJ) has a rich history that intertwines martial arts, philosophy, and personal development. Originating in Japan, the art of Jiu-Jitsu was adapted and popularized in Brazil by the Gracie family in the early 20th century. The Gracies, particularly Carlos and Helio, were instrumental in modifying traditional techniques to make them more effective for smaller individuals. This transformation emphasized leverage and technique over brute strength, making BJJ accessible to people of all shapes, sizes, and fitness levels. This foundational aspect has made BJJ a powerful tool for individuals seeking to build confidence and resilience in their lives.

As BJJ evolved, it gained recognition not only as a self-defense method but also as an avenue for personal growth and emotional regulation. Practitioners began to explore its psychological benefits, especially in relation to anxiety relief and stress management. The mat became a space where individuals could confront their fears, learn to manage their emotions, and develop mental toughness. This shift in focus has attracted a diverse array of participants, including professionals and sedentary individuals looking to improve their mental and physical well-being. The practice encourages self-reflection and fosters a sense of community, which is crucial for those overcoming trauma or seeking empowerment.

In addition to its emotional benefits, BJJ serves as a powerful mechanism for goal setting and personal growth. The structured nature of training allows individuals to set tangible objectives and track their progress over time. This goal-oriented mindset can be transformative, especially for those who have struggled with motivation or direction in their lives. As students progress through the belts, they not only acquire new skills but also learn valuable lessons about perseverance, discipline, and the importance of setting achievable goals. These experiences contribute to a stronger sense of self and the ability to face challenges both on and off the mats.

The history of Brazilian Jiu-Jitsu reflects its evolution into a multifaceted practice that addresses both physical and mental health needs. Its origins as a self-defense system have given way to a broader understanding of its role in fostering resilience, confidence, and personal empowerment. As individuals from various backgrounds continue to find solace and strength through BJJ, the art remains a beacon of hope and transformation for those striving to overcome personal struggles and achieve their fullest potential.

Core Principles of BJJ

The core principles of Brazilian Jiu-Jitsu (BJJ) are not just techniques and moves; they are foundational concepts that foster personal growth, resilience, and a deeper understanding of oneself. At the heart of BJJ lies the principle of leverage, which teaches practitioners how to use their body weight and positioning to overcome larger opponents. This fundamental concept transcends the mat, encouraging individuals, particularly those dealing with anxiety or self-doubt, to recognize that they can achieve success through strategy rather than sheer force. Learning to apply leverage in a physical context also mirrors the mental leverage one gains through practice and perseverance, reinforcing the idea that challenges can be tackled with the right mindset.

Another core principle is the adaptability that BJJ promotes. In training, practitioners often find themselves in unexpected positions or scenarios, requiring them to think critically and adjust their strategies in real time. This adaptability is crucial for personal development, especially for those who may feel overwhelmed by life's challenges. As individuals learn to navigate the dynamic landscape of BJJ, they also cultivate emotional intelligence, becoming more aware of their responses to stress and adversity. This heightened awareness fosters a sense of control, allowing practitioners to manage anxiety and build confidence in various aspects of their lives.

The principle of self-discipline is also integral to BJJ. Regular training instills a commitment to practice and improvement, encouraging individuals to set and achieve goals. This discipline is vital for those who may have previously struggled with sedentary lifestyles or low self-esteem. By establishing a routine and pushing through physical and mental barriers, practitioners develop a growth mindset that empowers them to pursue personal and professional goals with newfound determination. The journey of mastering techniques in BJJ serves as a metaphor for tackling life's obstacles, reinforcing the belief that consistent effort leads to progress.

Community plays a significant role in the BJJ experience. The supportive environment of a BJJ gym fosters connections among practitioners, promoting a sense of belonging and shared purpose. For many, this community provides an essential support network that can help in overcoming trauma and building mental toughness. Engaging with others who share similar challenges and aspirations fosters empathy and mutual respect, creating a safe space for individuals to express themselves and grow together. This sense of camaraderie is particularly empowering for women, encouraging them to embrace their strength and assertiveness in both BJJ and everyday life.

The principle of continuous learning is paramount in BJJ. The journey never truly ends; there is always something new to discover, whether it be a technique, a concept, or an approach to training. This commitment to lifelong learning fosters resilience, as practitioners learn to embrace failure as an opportunity for growth. For those facing personal challenges, this principle serves as a powerful reminder that setbacks are not the end but rather stepping stones to greater understanding and achievement. As individuals progress in their BJJ journey, they not only become more adept fighters but also more resilient, adaptable, and confident individuals ready to face life's challenges head-on.

BJJ as a Holistic Practice

Brazilian Jiu-Jitsu (BJJ) transcends the boundaries of a traditional martial art, emerging as a holistic practice that addresses both physical and mental well-being. For adults, especially those who may be new to physical activity, BJJ offers a unique pathway to enhance not only fitness but also emotional resilience. The practice integrates physical exertion with mental challenges, creating a space where individuals can confront their fears, manage anxiety, and cultivate stress relief. By engaging in BJJ, practitioners learn to navigate not only the dynamics of grappling but also the intricacies of their own emotional states.

The physical demands of BJJ promote a sense of accomplishment and empowerment, essential for building confidence and self-esteem. Each roll on the mat serves as a lesson in perseverance, teaching practitioners that progress comes through both success and failure. For those who may struggle with body image or self-worth, BJJ fosters an inclusive environment where individuals of all shapes and sizes can thrive. The collaborative nature of training allows for the development of camaraderie, reinforcing the idea that everyone has a place, which further bolsters personal confidence and encourages self-acceptance.

Emotional intelligence plays a pivotal role in the practice of BJJ, especially in coaching and mentorship. Coaches who prioritize emotional intelligence foster an atmosphere of trust and respect, enabling students to express their vulnerabilities and work through their challenges. This approach not only enhances the learning experience but also encourages practitioners to develop their own emotional regulation skills. As students learn to respond to the pressures of the mat, they simultaneously practice managing their emotions in real-world situations, equipping them with tools to handle stress and anxiety outside the dojo.

BJJ also serves as a powerful medium for overcoming trauma and building mental toughness. For individuals who have experienced trauma, the physicality of the practice can be both grounding and liberating. The discipline required in BJJ helps practitioners reclaim a sense of control over their bodies and minds. By facing fears in a supportive environment, individuals can process their experiences and develop resilience. The journey through BJJ becomes a metaphor for personal growth, illustrating that overcoming obstacles is possible through commitment and perseverance.

The principles of BJJ align seamlessly with personal growth and goal-setting. Practitioners are encouraged to set realistic, achievable goals, whether that be mastering a new technique or improving physical conditioning. This goal-oriented mindset not only fosters motivation but also provides a structured pathway for personal development. For women in particular, BJJ can be a transformative experience, promoting empowerment and self-defense skills while also providing a platform for emotional regulation. The holistic nature of BJJ nurtures a community where individuals can grow, heal, and thrive, illustrating that the journey from trauma to triumph is possible through the practice of Brazilian Jiu-Jitsu.

CHAPTER 3

Brazilian Jiu-Jitsu for Anxiety Relief and Stress Management

Physical Benefits of BJJ

Brazilian Jiu-Jitsu (BJJ) offers a multitude of physical benefits that extend beyond mere fitness. For adults, particularly those who may be overweight or sedentary, engaging in BJJ can serve as a transformative experience. The practice emphasizes cardiovascular endurance, strength, flexibility, and coordination. As practitioners roll on the mats, they engage in dynamic movements that elevate heart rates, promoting better overall cardiovascular health. This stimulation not only aids in weight loss but also enhances energy levels, making daily activities feel less burdensome.

17

One of the remarkable aspects of BJJ is its ability to build functional strength. Unlike traditional strength training that often isolates muscle groups, BJJ requires the use of multiple muscle groups in coordination. Practitioners learn to leverage their body weight and balance against their opponents, which develops core strength and improves muscle tone.

This functional approach to fitness is particularly beneficial for those who may have previously struggled with conventional workouts, as it introduces a playful yet challenging environment where progress is achievable and measurable.

Flexibility is another critical component of physical health that BJJ addresses. Many individuals, especially those who are new to physical activity, find that their range of motion is limited. BJJ techniques often involve stretching and maneuvering into various positions, which gradually increases flexibility over time. Enhanced flexibility not only improves performance on the mats but also reduces the risk of injuries in everyday life. This improvement can lead to greater freedom of movement, making routine tasks much easier and more enjoyable.

The physical demands of BJJ have a direct impact on mental well-being. The act of training, grappling, and sparring releases endorphins, which are the body's natural mood lifters. This biochemical response can significantly alleviate symptoms of anxiety and stress. For individuals seeking an outlet for their emotional struggles, BJJ provides a constructive way to channel negative energy into something positive. The combination of physical exertion and focused breathing techniques inherent in BJJ practice can serve as a form of moving meditation, promoting mental clarity and emotional regulation.

The community aspect of BJJ plays a crucial role in fostering physical and emotional resilience. As practitioners train together, they build bonds that contribute to a supportive environment. This camaraderie encourages individuals to push their limits, celebrate their progress, and hold each other accountable. For many, this sense of belonging can be a powerful antidote to feelings of isolation that often accompany trauma and anxiety. In essence, BJJ not only cultivates physical strength and fitness but also nurtures the spirit, making it a holistic approach to personal growth and empowerment.

Mental Benefits of BJJ

Mental benefits of Brazilian Jiu-Jitsu (BJJ) extend far beyond the physical aspects of the sport, offering profound effects on emotional well-being and psychological resilience. For adults, especially those who may be experiencing anxiety or stress, engaging in BJJ can serve as an effective means of managing these feelings. The immersive nature of BJJ requires focus and presence, which can help individuals shift their attention away from daily stressors and anxieties. By concentrating on techniques, movements, and strategies during training, practitioners often find a meditative quality to the practice, allowing for mental clarity and a reduction in feelings of overwhelm.

Building confidence and self-esteem is another significant mental benefit of BJJ. As students progress through the ranks, they gain tangible skills and achievements that foster a sense of accomplishment. This journey can be particularly impactful for those who may have felt marginalized or less capable in other areas of life. The supportive environment of a BJJ academy, where practitioners encourage each other, contributes to a culture of growth and empowerment. Achieving new belts or mastering a difficult technique can instill a stronger belief in one's abilities, translating into greater confidence both on and off the mats.

Integrating emotional intelligence into BJJ coaching can further enhance these mental benefits. Coaches who emphasize the importance of understanding emotions, both in themselves and in their students, create a more supportive learning environment. This approach encourages practitioners to recognize their emotional responses during training and competition, allowing them to develop better emotional regulation skills. By learning to navigate feelings of frustration, fear, or excitement, students can apply these lessons to everyday situations, improving their overall emotional resilience.

BJJ also plays a crucial role in overcoming trauma and building mental toughness. The practice often attracts individuals seeking to reclaim their power after difficult experiences. The discipline required in BJJ helps practitioners confront and work through their fears, both on the mats and in their personal lives. The physicality of training can serve as a healthy outlet for stress and emotional pain, while the community aspect fosters a sense of belonging and support. This powerful combination allows individuals to cultivate mental toughness and resilience, essential traits for navigating life's challenges.

Finally, BJJ can be a powerful tool for personal growth and goal setting. The structured nature of training and belt progression provides clear milestones for practitioners to strive for. This goal-oriented approach encourages individuals to set and achieve personal objectives, fostering a growth mindset. Furthermore, BJJ offers unique opportunities for female empowerment, as women increasingly find strength and confidence through training. The practice not only promotes physical fitness but also encourages emotional regulation, making it an effective means for individuals of all backgrounds to enhance their mental well-being and resilience.

Techniques for Managing Anxiety through BJJ

Techniques for managing anxiety through Brazilian Jiu-Jitsu (BJJ) are diverse and can be tailored to individual needs, making the practice a powerful tool for personal growth and emotional regulation. The physical nature of BJJ, which combines cardiovascular exercise with strength training, helps release endorphins, the body's natural mood lifters. This biochemical response is crucial for those struggling with anxiety, as it can lead to a reduction in stress and an improvement in overall mental health. Regular training not only fosters physical fitness but also creates a routine that can bring stability to daily life, alleviating feelings of uncertainty that often accompany anxiety.

Mindfulness is another technique that can be effectively integrated into BJJ practice. During training, practitioners are encouraged to focus on the present moment, paying attention to their breathing, movements, and the sensations in their bodies. This mindfulness approach helps individuals detach from anxious thoughts and feelings that may arise outside the dojo. By concentrating on the physical demands of BJJ, practitioners can cultivate a sense of calm and presence, which is beneficial for managing anxiety. Over time, this practice can extend beyond the mat, equipping individuals with tools to handle stress in various aspects of their lives.

Building confidence and self-esteem is a key benefit of practicing BJJ, which can significantly impact anxiety levels. As practitioners learn new techniques, gain skills, and achieve personal milestones, they experience a sense of accomplishment that boosts self-worth. This newfound confidence can transform how individuals perceive challenges, making them feel more equipped to face life's difficulties. Additionally, the supportive community often found within BJJ schools fosters connections and friendships, further enhancing emotional resilience and providing a network of encouragement that can help mitigate feelings of isolation associated with anxiety.

For those looking to integrate emotional intelligence into their BJJ practice, understanding one's emotional responses during training can lead to greater emotional regulation. Practicing BJJ often puts individuals in challenging situations that provoke anxiety, such as sparring with a partner or executing complex techniques.

Learning to navigate these emotions in a constructive manner helps individuals develop coping strategies that can be applied outside the dojo. Coaches who emphasize the importance of emotional awareness in their teaching can facilitate an environment where practitioners learn not only physical techniques but also how to manage their emotional states effectively.

For those looking to integrate emotional intelligence into their BJJ practice, understanding one's emotional responses during training can lead to greater emotional regulation. Practicing BJJ often puts individuals in challenging situations that provoke anxiety, such as sparring with a partner or executing complex techniques. Learning to navigate these emotions in a constructive manner helps individuals develop coping strategies that can be applied outside the dojo. Coaches who emphasize the importance of emotional awareness in their teaching can facilitate an environment where practitioners learn not only physical techniques but also how to manage their emotional states effectively.

CHAPTER 4

Building Confidence and Self-Esteem through BJJ

The Journey of Skill Acquisition

The journey of skill acquisition in Brazilian Jiu-Jitsu (BJJ) is a multifaceted process that goes beyond mere physical training. For adults, especially those dealing with anxiety, stress, or past trauma, this journey can serve as a powerful tool for personal growth and emotional regulation. As practitioners step onto the mat, they engage in a unique learning environment that fosters not only technical abilities but also mental resilience and confidence. This dual focus on physical and psychological development is essential for individuals looking to transform their lives through the practice of BJJ.

Initially, skill acquisition in BJJ involves understanding the fundamentals. New practitioners often find themselves overwhelmed by a multitude of techniques and concepts. However, this stage is crucial for building a solid foundation. Instructors guide students through basic movements, helping them develop essential motor skills and body awareness. This process requires patience and consistency, which are vital qualities that transfer to other areas of life, especially for those who may have experienced setbacks or challenges. The ability to embrace the learning curve can significantly enhance self-esteem and create a sense of achievement.

As practitioners progress, they encounter various obstacles that test their mental toughness. Sparring sessions, in particular, challenge individuals to apply what they've learned under pressure. This experience can be a powerful metaphor for life's challenges, helping students to develop resilience. Each defeat on the mat teaches valuable lessons about perseverance, humility, and the importance of maintaining a growth mindset. For those struggling with anxiety or self-doubt, facing these challenges head-on can lead to breakthroughs in confidence and emotional regulation, equipping them with tools to manage stress outside the dojo.

Moreover, the social aspect of BJJ plays a significant role in the journey of skill acquisition. Practitioners often form strong bonds with their training partners, creating a supportive community that fosters growth. This environment encourages open communication and emotional intelligence, essential components for effective coaching and personal development. As students learn to work with others, they also learn the importance of empathy, teamwork, and mutual respect. These social dynamics not only enhance the training experience but also empower individuals, particularly women, to assert themselves and cultivate a sense of belonging.

Ultimately, the journey of skill acquisition in BJJ is a holistic process that integrates physical, mental, and emotional growth. Each step taken on the mat contributes to a larger narrative of overcoming adversity and building resilience. For adults seeking transformation, BJJ offers a pathway to reclaim control over their lives, fostering a sense of empowerment and purpose. By embracing this journey, practitioners can harness their experiences in BJJ to set meaningful goals and achieve personal growth, making it a valuable tool for navigating the complexities of life.

Overcoming Challenges on the Mat

Overcoming challenges on the mat is an integral part of the Brazilian Jiu-Jitsu experience, particularly for those who may be grappling with personal struggles such as anxiety, low self-esteem, or trauma. As participants engage in this physically demanding sport, they confront not only their opponents but also their own limitations and fears. Each roll on the mat becomes an opportunity for self-discovery, where practitioners learn to navigate discomfort, embrace vulnerability, and develop resilience. The unique environment of Brazilian Jiu-Jitsu fosters a sense of community, offering support and encouragement as individuals work through their personal challenges.

For many, the physicality of BJJ serves as a powerful mechanism for stress relief. The act of grappling requires intense focus, pushing aside external worries and anxieties. Participants find themselves immersed in the moment, where the only thing that matters is the next movement, the next escape, or the next submission. This mindfulness aspect not only alleviates stress but also promotes emotional regulation. As practitioners learn to control their breathing and reactions during intense situations on the mat, they simultaneously cultivate skills that can be applied off the mat, leading to improved emotional intelligence and coping strategies in everyday life.

Building confidence and self-esteem is another critical benefit of overcoming challenges in BJJ. For those who have struggled with feelings of inadequacy or fear of failure, the journey through Brazilian Jiu-Jitsu offers a transformative experience. Many individuals find that with each small victory — whether it's mastering a new technique or successfully rolling with a more experienced partner — they gain a deeper sense of self-worth. Over time, these incremental successes accumulate, reshaping one's self-image and bolstering resilience. This newfound confidence extends beyond the mat, empowering individuals to set and pursue personal goals in various aspects of their lives.

Brazilian Jiu-Jitsu has proven to be an effective tool for those overcoming trauma. The practice encourages individuals to confront their fears and insecurities in a safe environment, allowing them to process past experiences while cultivating mental toughness. The act of grappling itself can be metaphorical for wrestling with one's own demons, providing a pathway to healing. Instructors who integrate emotional intelligence into their coaching can further enhance this experience, offering tailored guidance that acknowledges each student's unique background and challenges, thus fostering a supportive atmosphere conducive to growth and recovery.

BJJ serves as a platform for personal growth and empowerment, particularly for women who may have faced societal challenges related to their self-image or assertiveness. The sport not only builds physical strength but also encourages emotional resilience, helping individuals learn to advocate for themselves and assert their boundaries. Through the journey of training, participants develop a sense of agency and ownership over their bodies and experiences. By embracing the challenges faced on the mat, practitioners not only achieve physical milestones but also cultivate a deeper understanding of themselves, paving the way for triumph over adversity in all areas of life.

The Role of Community and Support

The journey through trauma towards triumph is often a solitary path, but Brazilian Jiu-Jitsu (BJJ) offers a unique opportunity for individuals to find community and support in their healing process. The shared experience of training creates a sense of belonging that is crucial for mental resilience. In BJJ academies, practitioners come together, regardless of their backgrounds, to work towards common goals, fostering an environment where connection and camaraderie flourish. This supportive atmosphere helps individuals feel less isolated in their struggles, allowing for open discussions about mental health, anxiety, and personal challenges.

Community support in BJJ extends beyond the physical training; it encompasses emotional and social dimensions that are vital for personal growth.

Practitioners often form deep bonds with their teammates, cultivating an environment where vulnerability is welcomed and encouraged. These relationships can provide a safety net for individuals dealing with anxiety or self-esteem issues, as they can share experiences and strategies for coping. The mentorship from more experienced practitioners also plays a significant role, as they can offer guidance and reassurance to newcomers navigating their own challenges.

Moreover, BJJ serves as a platform for building confidence and self-esteem, particularly for those who may have felt marginalized or insecure in other areas of their lives. The act of learning and mastering techniques fosters a sense of accomplishment that translates into greater self-worth. As students progress, they gain not only physical skills but also the mental fortitude to face adversities outside the mat. This newfound confidence can lead to an enhanced ability to manage stress, as individuals learn to confront their fears in a safe and supportive environment.

Emotional intelligence is another crucial aspect of community support in BJJ. Coaches and teammates often engage in discussions about emotional regulation and resilience, creating a culture that prioritizes mental well-being alongside physical prowess. By integrating emotional intelligence into training, practitioners learn to recognize their own emotions and those of others, enhancing their ability to connect and empathize. This awareness is particularly empowering for women in BJJ, as it cultivates a sense of agency and self-regulation, crucial for overcoming societal pressures and personal trauma.

The role of community and support in BJJ cannot be overstated. It transforms the experience of grappling with personal challenges into a collective journey toward growth and healing. As individuals come together to share their stories and strengths, they create an encouraging network that amplifies the benefits of BJJ in overcoming trauma and enhancing mental resilience. In this way, Brazilian Jiu-Jitsu becomes not just a sport but a vital tool for personal development, inviting everyone—regardless of their starting point—to embrace the journey from trauma to triumph.

CHAPTER 5

Integrating Emotional Intelligence in BJJ Coaching

Defining Emotional Intelligence in Sports

Emotional intelligence in sports refers to the ability to recognize, understand, and manage one's own emotions while also being aware of and influencing the emotions of others. In the context of Brazilian Jiu-Jitsu (BJJ), this multifaceted skill set is crucial not only for performance on the mat but also for personal development and emotional well-being. Athletes who cultivate emotional intelligence can navigate the challenges of training and competition more effectively, leading to enhanced resilience and overall mental health.

One key aspect of emotional intelligence is self-awareness, which allows practitioners to identify their emotional responses to various situations. For those engaging in BJJ, whether new to the sport or seasoned practitioners, understanding triggers such as anxiety or frustration during sparring sessions can be transformative. By recognizing these emotions, individuals can develop strategies to manage them, fostering a more focused and confident approach to their training and competition.

Empathy, another component of emotional intelligence, plays a significant role in BJJ. As a martial art that emphasizes respect and understanding of one's training partners, practitioners learn to read the emotions of others, which can enhance teamwork and camaraderie. Developing this empathic connection not only improves the training environment but also empowers individuals to support one another in overcoming personal challenges, such as anxiety or low self-esteem. This collective emotional resilience creates a supportive community where everyone can thrive.

Emotional regulation, a vital skill within emotional intelligence, is particularly important in high-pressure environments like competitive BJJ. Athletes often face intense emotions that can impact their performance, such as fear of failure or the stress of competition. By honing the ability to regulate these emotions, practitioners can maintain composure and focus, ultimately improving their chances of success. This skill is invaluable not just in sports but in daily life, as it translates into better stress management and overall emotional health.

Finally, integrating emotional intelligence into BJJ coaching can significantly enhance the experience for both instructors and students. Coaches who understand and apply principles of emotional intelligence create a more engaging and supportive atmosphere, facilitating personal growth and goal setting. By fostering an environment where emotional awareness and regulation are prioritized, coaches can help individuals—especially those facing trauma or seeking empowerment—build the mental toughness required to navigate life's challenges, both on and off the mat.

Coaching Strategies for Emotional Awareness

Coaching strategies that emphasize emotional awareness are crucial for practitioners of Brazilian Jiu-Jitsu, particularly for adults navigating anxiety, stress, and self-esteem challenges. An effective approach begins with creating a safe and supportive environment where individuals feel comfortable expressing their emotions. Coaches should encourage open dialogues about feelings before, during, and after training sessions. This practice not only fosters a sense of community but also helps individuals recognize and articulate their emotional states, facilitating a deeper connection between physical practice and emotional well-being.

Incorporating mindfulness techniques into training can significantly enhance emotional awareness. Coaches can introduce breathing exercises and meditation practices before or after sessions, allowing participants to center themselves and tune into their feelings. By focusing on the present moment, individuals can better understand their emotional responses to stressors, both on and off the mat. This practice of mindfulness can help reduce anxiety, improve concentration, and increase overall emotional resilience, which is particularly beneficial for those dealing with trauma or seeking personal growth.

Another effective strategy involves using role-playing scenarios and situational drills that simulate high-pressure environments. These exercises can help students confront their emotional reactions to challenges, such as fear of failure or feelings of inadequacy. By providing a structured setting to explore these emotions, coaches can guide participants in developing coping strategies and emotional regulation techniques. This experiential learning is vital for building mental toughness and can empower practitioners, particularly women, to navigate their emotional landscapes with confidence and assertiveness.

Setting personal goals within the context of BJJ training can also enhance emotional awareness. Coaches should encourage students to define their objectives, whether they focus on skill development, competition, or personal growth. By regularly revisiting these goals, individuals can reflect on their emotional journey and recognize how their emotions influence their progress. This reflection fosters a greater sense of accountability and self-awareness, allowing practitioners to celebrate their achievements and learn from setbacks, ultimately reinforcing their emotional resilience.

Integrating emotional intelligence into BJJ coaching can transform the training experience. Coaches who model emotional awareness and regulation can inspire students to adopt similar practices. By teaching athletes to recognize their emotions and the emotions of others, they can cultivate empathy and understanding within the training environment. This not only enhances the overall experience but also empowers individuals to leverage their emotional insights for personal development. As students learn to navigate their emotions more effectively, they become better equipped to handle life's challenges outside the dojo, further promoting mental resilience and emotional well-being.

Creating a Supportive Training Environment

Creating a supportive training environment is essential for fostering growth and resilience in practitioners of Brazilian Jiu-Jitsu, especially for adults who may be new to the sport or returning after a period of inactivity. A welcoming atmosphere encourages participation from individuals of all backgrounds, including those who may feel anxious or uncertain about stepping onto the mat. Establishing a culture of inclusivity is critical; it allows practitioners to focus on their personal growth without the fear of judgment. This supportive setting can significantly enhance their experience, making the journey from trauma to triumph a more attainable goal.

The physical space where training occurs plays a vital role in creating a supportive environment. Mats should be clean and well-maintained, with adequate space for everyone to practice safely. Additionally, the layout should promote interaction, allowing practitioners to engage with one another, share experiences, and build camaraderie. Lighting and ventilation should also be considered to make the environment comfortable. This attention to the physical aspects of the training space contributes to a sense of belonging, especially for those who might feel out of place due to their body type or fitness level.

Coaching styles and communication techniques are pivotal in establishing a supportive training culture. Instructors should prioritize emotional intelligence, recognizing the diverse backgrounds and experiences of their students. This means being attentive to the individual needs of practitioners, offering encouragement, and providing constructive feedback. Coaches can foster an environment where mistakes are viewed as learning opportunities rather than failures. This approach builds confidence and self-esteem, allowing students to embrace challenges and push through their limitations.

Peer support is another critical component of a nurturing training environment. Encouraging students to partner with different training partners helps them develop social skills and creates a sense of community. When practitioners support each other, they cultivate a network that promotes emotional regulation and resilience. This is especially important for individuals who use BJJ as a tool for overcoming trauma, as building trust with fellow practitioners can enhance their overall mental well-being. Celebrating each other's successes, no matter how small, reinforces a supportive atmosphere where everyone feels valued.

Finally, integrating goal-setting into the training process can empower practitioners and provide a clear path for personal growth. Instructors should encourage students to define their own objectives, whether they relate to technique mastery, fitness improvements, or emotional healing. By framing these goals within a supportive context, practitioners can measure their progress and celebrate achievements together. This not only enhances individual resilience but also strengthens the bonds within the training community, ultimately making Brazilian Jiu-Jitsu a transformative experience for all involved.

CHAPTER 6

The Role of BJJ in Overcoming Trauma and Building Mental Toughness

Personal Stories of Triumph

In the journey from trauma to triumph, personal stories often serve as powerful reminders of human resilience and the transformative potential of Brazilian Jiu-Jitsu (BJJ). One remarkable example is that of Sarah, a former corporate professional who struggled with anxiety and self-doubt. After experiencing a significant life event that left her feeling overwhelmed, she turned to BJJ not just as a physical outlet but as a means of reclaiming her sense of self. Through the rigorous training and supportive community of her dojo, Sarah gradually learned to navigate her anxiety. Each roll on the mat became a metaphor for her struggles, teaching her that perseverance and technique could overcome feelings of helplessness.

Another inspiring story comes from Mark, who battled obesity and sedentary habits for years. Overwhelmed by societal pressures and personal insecurities, he found it difficult to engage in traditional fitness programs. However, BJJ offered him a unique environment where he could focus on skill development rather than just weight loss. With each technique learned and every sparring session, Mark not only shed pounds but also built a newfound confidence and self-esteem. His journey illustrates how BJJ can be a gateway to personal growth, enabling individuals to set and achieve goals they once thought impossible.

The impact of BJJ extends beyond physical transformation; it also fosters emotional intelligence. Take the case of Linda, a coach who integrated emotional regulation techniques within her BJJ classes. By sharing her own experiences of overcoming trauma, she created a safe space for her students, particularly women, to express vulnerabilities and build resilience. Linda's approach emphasizes the importance of emotional awareness and regulation, illustrating how BJJ can empower individuals to confront their fears and develop a greater sense of agency in their lives.

Another powerful narrative comes from Jason, a veteran who sought solace in BJJ after returning from service. The physical demands of the sport helped him channel his anxiety and PTSD into something productive. Through the camaraderie of his training partners, Jason found a support system that enabled him to process his experiences and rebuild his mental toughness. His story highlights how BJJ can serve as a therapeutic outlet, allowing individuals to confront and overcome their past traumas in a constructive manner.

Finally, consider the journey of Maria, who initially joined a BJJ class seeking self-defense skills but discovered much more. Her experience in the dojo transformed her understanding of empowerment and personal growth. As she progressed in her training, Maria became a mentor to other women, encouraging them to embrace their strength and resilience. Her story exemplifies how BJJ can cultivate a sense of community and support, fostering an environment where individuals can thrive emotionally and mentally while pursuing their goals.

BJJ as a Therapeutic Tool

Brazilian Jiu-Jitsu (BJJ) serves as more than just a physical discipline; it is increasingly recognized as a powerful therapeutic tool that can facilitate healing and personal growth. For adults grappling with anxiety and stress, the practice of BJJ provides a unique outlet for emotional release. The structured environment of the dojo encourages individuals to confront their fears in a controlled setting, enabling them to develop coping mechanisms that can be applied outside the mat. The combination of physical exertion and mental focus fosters a sense of calm, allowing practitioners to manage their anxiety levels more effectively while promoting overall mental well-being.

Building confidence and self-esteem is another vital aspect of BJJ that resonates deeply with practitioners from all walks of life. As individuals learn and master new techniques, they experience a sense of accomplishment that translates into increased self-assuredness. This growth is particularly significant for those who may have struggled with self-image or feelings of inadequacy. The supportive community within BJJ fosters camaraderie and encouragement, allowing newcomers and seasoned practitioners alike to share their journeys. This environment not only builds physical skills but also reinforces a positive self-identity, empowering individuals to tackle life's challenges with newfound resilience.

Emotional intelligence plays a critical role in the coaching and practice of BJJ. Coaches who incorporate principles of emotional awareness into their training can help students navigate their feelings more effectively, enhancing the overall learning experience. By fostering an environment where emotions are acknowledged and discussed, practitioners can develop greater empathy and understanding, both on and off the mat. This integration of emotional intelligence not only improves interpersonal skills but also equips individuals to handle conflict and stress in more constructive ways, fostering healthier relationships in their personal and professional lives.

For those overcoming trauma, BJJ provides a framework for building mental toughness and resilience. The act of grappling with an opponent is not just a physical battle; it mirrors the internal struggles many face after experiencing trauma. Through consistent practice, individuals learn to confront discomfort and adversity, gradually desensitizing themselves to past emotional pain. This process of exposure, coupled with the supportive community in BJJ, allows individuals to reclaim their narratives and cultivate a sense of empowerment. The journey through BJJ becomes a metaphor for overcoming obstacles, reinforcing the belief that individuals can rise above their circumstances.

Finally, BJJ serves as a catalyst for personal growth and goal setting. The structured progression of belts and techniques provides clear milestones that practitioners can strive to achieve, instilling a sense of purpose and direction. For overweight or sedentary individuals, setting and accomplishing fitness-related goals within the context of BJJ can lead to transformative changes in both body and mind. Additionally, for women, BJJ offers a unique platform for empowerment, encouraging emotional regulation and self-defense skills. The practice fosters an environment where female practitioners can build confidence, assertiveness, and resilience, ultimately leading to a more balanced and fulfilled life. Through these avenues, BJJ emerges as a comprehensive therapeutic tool that transcends mere physicality, guiding individuals towards holistic well-being and personal triumph.

Developing Mental Toughness through Practice

Developing mental toughness through practice is a fundamental aspect of Brazilian Jiu-Jitsu, serving both as a skill set and a mindset that can be cultivated over time. For adults, particularly those who may feel overwhelmed by anxiety or stress, engaging in BJJ offers an effective way to confront challenges head-on. The practice itself is a microcosm of life's struggles; each roll or sparring session presents an opportunity to face discomfort, push through mental barriers, and develop resilience. As practitioners learn to navigate these physical and emotional challenges, they cultivate a sense of mental toughness that extends beyond the mats and into their daily lives.

Regular practice in Brazilian Jiu-Jitsu provides a structured environment where individuals can confront their fears and insecurities. Over time, as they face opponents of varying skill levels and sizes, practitioners learn that they can endure discomfort and overcome obstacles. This process fosters a unique form of self-confidence that is built not just on physical ability but also on the mental fortitude developed through perseverance. For many, especially those who may have struggled with self-esteem, the realization that they can push through tough situations in training translates into a renewed belief in their capabilities outside the gym.

Moreover, the nature of BJJ encourages emotional intelligence. As practitioners engage in sparring and technique drills, they learn to read their opponents, anticipate moves, and respond to challenges in real-time. This interaction requires a level of self-awareness and empathy, fostering both personal growth and an understanding of others. For those who have experienced trauma, this aspect of BJJ can be particularly empowering, as it teaches individuals to recognize their emotions and react constructively. By integrating emotional intelligence into their practice, students can better manage their reactions to stress and anxiety, ultimately reinforcing their mental toughness.

Goal setting is another key component in developing mental toughness through Brazilian Jiu-Jitsu. Each belt promotion, competition, or personal milestone offers a tangible objective that practitioners can strive for. Setting these goals creates a roadmap for growth, allowing individuals to track their progress and celebrate achievements along the way. For those who may have previously felt stagnant or unmotivated, the discipline and structure of BJJ provide a powerful framework for personal development. This journey not only enhances physical skills but also instills a sense of purpose and direction, further solidifying mental resilience.

Finally, the inclusive nature of the BJJ community plays a significant role in fostering mental toughness. Practitioners, regardless of their background or fitness level, are welcomed and encouraged, creating a supportive environment for all. This sense of camaraderie helps individuals feel less isolated in their struggles, promoting a collective journey towards self-improvement. Women, in particular, can find empowerment through BJJ, as they learn to assert themselves and develop emotional regulation in a traditionally male-dominated sport. By building a strong support network and engaging in a practice that emphasizes growth and resilience, individuals can transform their experiences from trauma into triumph, emerging with enhanced mental toughness that benefits every aspect of their lives.

CHAPTER 7

BJJ as a Tool for Personal Growth and Goal Setting

Setting Realistic Goals in BJJ

Setting realistic goals in Brazilian Jiu-Jitsu (BJJ) is essential for anyone embarking on this journey, particularly for adults who may be new to the sport or returning after a long hiatus. The nature of BJJ can be intimidating, especially for those who are overweight or sedentary, but establishing attainable goals can foster a sense of achievement and encourage consistent participation. It is crucial to recognize that progress in BJJ is often nonlinear; setting small, realistic milestones allows practitioners to celebrate victories along the way, which can significantly boost motivation and enjoyment of the practice.

For individuals seeking anxiety relief and stress management through BJJ, setting specific and measurable goals is key. Instead of aiming for an abstract outcome, such as becoming a black belt, practitioners could focus on mastering a particular technique or attending classes a certain number of times per week. These smaller, concrete objectives not only provide clear targets but also create opportunities for reflection and self-assessment. As practitioners achieve these goals, they can build confidence and reduce anxiety, reinforcing the positive mental health benefits of their BJJ training.

Building confidence and self-esteem is another vital aspect of goal setting in BJJ. Many adults may feel self-conscious or doubt their abilities, especially in a martial art that emphasizes technique and skill. By setting realistic goals, such as rolling with a partner of similar experience or successfully executing a submission in sparring, individuals can gradually enhance their self-efficacy. Each small success contributes to a stronger sense of self-worth, which is particularly empowering for women in the sport. This process of setting and achieving goals can act as a powerful catalyst for personal growth and resilience.

Emotional intelligence plays a significant role in BJJ coaching and goal setting. Coaches should encourage students to articulate their goals and understand the emotional aspects of their training journey. This collaborative approach allows practitioners to set goals that resonate with their personal experiences and aspirations. For instance, a student may want to work on their ability to manage frustration during training sessions. By integrating emotional regulation techniques into their practice, they can create a supportive environment that fosters personal development and mental toughness.

Finally, the role of BJJ in overcoming trauma and fostering personal growth cannot be overstated. Setting realistic goals provides a structured framework that allows individuals to confront their fears and past experiences in a safe environment. As practitioners work through their goals, they build resilience and mental toughness, empowering them to navigate challenges both on and off the mat. By recognizing the importance of goal setting in their BJJ practice, individuals can harness the transformative power of the art to cultivate a healthier mindset, improve overall well-being, and achieve a sense of triumph in their lives.

The Process of Self-Discovery

The process of self-discovery is a transformative journey that often unfolds within the practice of Brazilian Jiu-Jitsu (BJJ). For many individuals, particularly those who may have experienced trauma or struggle with anxiety, engaging in BJJ provides a unique opportunity to explore their identities and uncover hidden strengths. As practitioners step onto the mat, they confront not only their physical limitations but also their emotional barriers. This confrontation leads to moments of introspection, where individuals can reflect on their motivations, fears, and aspirations, ultimately fostering a deeper understanding of themselves.

One significant aspect of self-discovery in BJJ is the development of mental resilience. As students progress in their training, they face challenges that require problem-solving and adaptability. Each roll on the mat serves as a microcosm of life's larger challenges, teaching practitioners how to navigate adversity and setbacks. This process cultivates a growth mindset, allowing individuals to redefine their self-image and shift their perspective on failure. The lessons learned during sparring sessions become invaluable tools for tackling external stressors, reinforcing the idea that resilience is not merely a trait but a skill that can be honed.

Moreover, BJJ promotes confidence and self-esteem through tangible achievements. The journey from beginner to advanced practitioner is marked by milestones such as earning stripes and belts. These achievements serve not only as recognition of hard work but also as reminders of the progress made. For those who may have struggled with feelings of inadequacy or low self-worth, this recognition can be life-changing. As practitioners gain confidence in their abilities on the mat, they often find that this newfound self-assurance extends to other areas of their lives, enhancing their professional and personal interactions.

Emotional intelligence plays a crucial role in the self-discovery process within BJJ. The sport emphasizes the importance of understanding one's own emotions and those of others, particularly during training and competition. Practitioners learn to regulate their emotional responses, which is vital for maintaining composure in high-pressure situations. This emotional regulation not only benefits individuals in their BJJ practice but also translates to improved interpersonal relationships and workplace dynamics. By integrating emotional intelligence into their training, practitioners sharpen their ability to empathize, communicate, and collaborate, fostering a holistic approach to personal growth.

Brazilian Jiu-Jitsu serves as a powerful tool for personal growth and goal setting. The practice encourages individuals to set specific, measurable goals, whether related to fitness, technique, or competition. This goal-oriented mindset instills a sense of purpose and direction, guiding practitioners through their self-discovery journeys. Additionally, BJJ offers a supportive community that empowers individuals, particularly women, to embrace their strength and resilience. As practitioners navigate the complexities of their emotional landscapes and redefine their identities, they emerge not only as skilled martial artists but also as more self-aware and empowered individuals ready to face life's challenges head-on.

Applying BJJ Principles to Everyday Life

Applying the principles of Brazilian Jiu-Jitsu (BJJ) to everyday life can significantly enhance mental resilience and personal growth. The core tenets of BJJ, including adaptability, problem-solving, and perseverance, can be transformative for individuals facing various challenges, from anxiety and stress to issues of self-esteem and trauma. By embracing these principles outside the mat, practitioners can cultivate a mindset that promotes emotional regulation and personal empowerment, enriching their daily experiences.

One essential principle of BJJ is adaptability. On the mat, practitioners learn to respond fluidly to their opponents' movements, adjusting strategies in real-time. This skill translates well into everyday situations, where adaptability can help individuals navigate unexpected obstacles or changes. For professionals facing workplace stress, being able to pivot and adjust to new demands can alleviate anxiety and enhance performance. Similarly, for those managing personal challenges, adopting a flexible mindset fosters resilience, allowing for better coping mechanisms in the face of adversity.

Problem-solving is another critical aspect of BJJ that can be applied to daily life. Each training session presents a series of challenges that require strategic thinking and innovative solutions. This approach encourages a proactive attitude toward life's difficulties. When faced with problems, whether they relate to health, relationships, or career, individuals can draw on their BJJ training to break down issues into manageable components, identify potential solutions, and implement them with confidence. This method not only builds mental toughness but also reinforces the belief that challenges can be overcome through thoughtful action.

Perseverance, a cornerstone of BJJ, teaches practitioners the value of persistence in the face of failure. In training, individuals often encounter setbacks, yet the commitment to keep trying leads to growth and improvement. This principle is particularly relevant for those dealing with trauma or self-doubt, as it instills a sense of hope and determination. By embracing the idea that progress is often non-linear, individuals can approach their personal goals with a more forgiving perspective, allowing for setbacks without losing sight of their overall aspirations.

Furthermore, BJJ promotes emotional intelligence, a vital tool for personal and professional interactions. Through grappling, individuals learn to read their opponents' emotions and reactions, fostering empathy and understanding. This heightened awareness can be beneficial in everyday life, enhancing communication skills and relationships. For those seeking to build confidence and self-esteem, engaging in BJJ provides a supportive environment where emotional regulation is practiced, empowering individuals to express themselves authentically and assertively.

Ultimately, the lessons learned through Brazilian Jiu-Jitsu extend far beyond the mat. By internalizing the principles of adaptability, problem-solving, perseverance, and emotional intelligence, individuals can effectively navigate the complexities of daily life. These skills not only contribute to overcoming challenges associated with anxiety and trauma but also promote personal growth and empowerment. As practitioners apply these BJJ principles to their lives, they embark on a transformative journey from trauma to triumph, building the mental resilience necessary to thrive in a complex world.

CHAPTER 8

Female Empowerment and Emotional Regulation in BJJ

The Importance of Female Representation in BJJ

The representation of women in Brazilian Jiu-Jitsu (BJJ) is not merely a matter of equality; it is fundamental to the growth and evolution of the sport. Female athletes bring unique perspectives and experiences that enrich the practice of BJJ. Their participation challenges traditional gender roles and inspires both men and women to see the art as inclusive and accessible. When women are visible in leadership positions, coaching roles, and competition, it sets a precedent that encourages more individuals, especially those who may feel marginalized, to engage with BJJ. This shift is vital for cultivating a community that values diversity and inclusivity, ultimately benefiting everyone involved.

For adults grappling with anxiety and stress, the presence of female role models in BJJ can be particularly impactful. Women who have successfully navigated their own challenges through the sport serve as living proof of its transformative power. Their stories resonate with those who may feel overwhelmed by life's pressures. These role models demonstrate that BJJ is not solely for the traditionally athletic or fit; it is a practice that can be embraced by anyone seeking empowerment and personal growth. By seeing women excel in BJJ, newcomers may feel encouraged to step onto the mat, knowing that they are part of a welcoming and supportive environment.

Building confidence and self-esteem is a core benefit of practicing BJJ, and female representation plays a crucial role in this process. Women who train in BJJ experience significant growth in their self-assurance, often overcoming societal pressures that dictate how they should behave or what they can achieve. This empowerment is magnified when they see other women succeeding in the sport. The journey of female practitioners fosters a collective resilience, where each woman's triumph helps to uplift others. This dynamic not only promotes individual confidence but strengthens the community, creating a network of support that can be particularly beneficial for those who may struggle with self-worth.

Finally, the role of BJJ in personal growth and goal setting is further enriched by female representation. Women involved in the sport often set ambitious goals, whether in competition or personal development. Their achievements can inspire others to adopt a similar mindset, emphasizing that BJJ is a powerful tool for anyone looking to overcome obstacles and pursue their aspirations. In a world where women are frequently underrepresented in various domains, their visibility in BJJ not only empowers them but also encourages a broader conversation about the importance of inclusivity. By embracing female representation, BJJ becomes a catalyst for change, fostering a culture where everyone, regardless of gender, can thrive and transform their lives.

BJJ as a Platform for Empowerment

Brazilian Jiu-Jitsu (BJJ) serves as a powerful platform for empowerment, particularly for individuals navigating mental health challenges such as anxiety and stress. The practice of BJJ encourages participants to confront their fears and overcome them in a controlled environment. This martial art is not solely about physical prowess; it emphasizes strategy, technique, and mental fortitude. As practitioners learn to grapple with opponents, they frequently find that they are also grappling with their own inner turmoil. Each roll on the mat becomes an opportunity to face and manage anxiety, allowing individuals to cultivate resilience and find relief from daily stressors.

Building confidence and self-esteem is another significant benefit of engaging with Brazilian Jiu-Jitsu. For many, the journey begins with feeling out of place or intimidated by the skill level of others. However, as individuals commit to training, they gradually improve their techniques and gain recognition for their progress. The sense of accomplishment that arises from mastering a new skill or successfully executing a technique fosters a growing sense of self-worth. This newfound confidence often transcends the mat, influencing other aspects of life, including personal relationships and professional endeavors, thereby reinforcing the idea that empowerment through BJJ extends well beyond physical training.

Integrating emotional intelligence into BJJ coaching further enhances the empowerment experience. Coaches who understand the psychological aspects of their students can create a supportive environment where practitioners feel safe to express their emotions and vulnerabilities. This approach facilitates open dialogue about feelings related to training and personal challenges, promoting a culture of empathy and understanding. By fostering emotional intelligence, coaches help their students develop not only their grappling abilities but also their capacity to navigate life's challenges with greater emotional awareness and resilience.

BJJ also plays a significant role in overcoming trauma and building mental toughness. For individuals who have experienced trauma, the physicality of BJJ can serve as a therapeutic outlet. The act of engaging in a physical confrontation can help reclaim a sense of agency and control. Techniques learned in BJJ encourage practitioners to remain calm under pressure, a skill that translates to improved coping mechanisms in everyday life. As individuals learn to trust their bodies and instincts through BJJ, they gradually build the mental toughness required to face adversities head-on.

Brazilian Jiu-Jitsu is a valuable tool for personal growth and goal setting. The structured nature of training provides a clear pathway for setting and achieving goals, whether they are related to fitness, technique, or competition. Each milestone reached serves as a reminder of one's capabilities and potential. Additionally, BJJ fosters a sense of community where individuals can support one another in their journeys, further reinforcing the idea of empowerment. For women, in particular, BJJ offers a unique platform for empowerment and emotional regulation, enabling them to navigate challenges confidently and assertively. In this way, BJJ becomes a transformative practice that not only builds physical strength but also cultivates a resilient mindset essential for triumphing over life's obstacles.

Strategies for Emotional Regulation in Training

Emotional regulation is a critical skill for practitioners of Brazilian Jiu-Jitsu (BJJ), particularly for adults navigating challenges such as anxiety, stress, and self-esteem issues. Training in BJJ can evoke a range of emotions, from frustration to exhilaration. By implementing specific strategies for emotional regulation, individuals can enhance their training experience and foster personal growth. These strategies not only facilitate better performance on the mat but also contribute to overall mental resilience.

One effective strategy for emotional regulation is mindfulness. Practicing mindfulness during training helps individuals become more aware of their feelings and physical sensations without judgment. This awareness allows practitioners to identify their emotional triggers, whether it be the pressure of competition or the challenges of learning new techniques. By focusing on the present moment and accepting emotions as they arise, individuals can reduce anxiety and improve their capacity to respond to stressors in a calm and composed manner. Mindfulness exercises, such as deep breathing and visualization, can be incorporated into warm-ups or cooldowns to reinforce this practice.

Another strategy is the use of positive self-talk. Negative thoughts can hinder performance and contribute to feelings of inadequacy, especially for those who may struggle with self-esteem. By consciously replacing negative self-talk with affirmations of strength and resilience, practitioners can cultivate a more positive mindset. For example, repeating phrases like "I am capable" or "I can learn from my mistakes" can help shift focus from fear of failure to a growth-oriented perspective. This mental shift not only enhances confidence but also encourages perseverance in the face of challenges, making the training environment more supportive and empowering.

Setting clear and achievable goals is also vital for emotional regulation in BJJ. Individuals can break down their long-term aspirations into smaller, manageable objectives that can be tracked and celebrated. This process fosters a sense of accomplishment, which boosts self-esteem and motivation. Whether the goal is to master a specific technique, improve physical fitness, or compete in a tournament, having a clear roadmap provides direction and purpose. Furthermore, achieving these incremental goals reinforces the belief that progress is attainable, which is crucial for those overcoming past trauma or anxiety.

Fostering a supportive community within the BJJ environment can greatly enhance emotional regulation. Building connections with training partners and coaches creates a network of encouragement and accountability. Sharing experiences, challenges, and victories helps normalize the emotional ups and downs associated with training. For many, especially those who may feel isolated due to anxiety or trauma, this sense of belonging can be transformative. Supportive relationships encourage individuals to express their feelings, seek help when needed, and celebrate each other's progress, reinforcing the idea that emotional regulation is a shared journey.

In conclusion, the strategies for emotional regulation in BJJ—mindfulness, positive self-talk, goal setting, and community support—are invaluable tools for individuals seeking to enhance their training experience and personal growth. These techniques not only improve performance on the mat but also contribute significantly to building mental resilience, overcoming trauma, and fostering a sense of empowerment. By incorporating these strategies into their practice, practitioners can navigate their emotional landscapes with greater ease, ultimately transforming their training into a powerful vehicle for healing and self-improvement.

CHAPTER 9

Creating a Resilient Mindset

Understanding the Growth Mindset

Understanding the growth mindset is essential for anyone looking to harness the transformative power of Brazilian Jiu-Jitsu (BJJ). This concept, popularized by psychologist Carol Dweck, focuses on the belief that abilities and intelligence can be developed through dedication and hard work. For adults, particularly those facing challenges such as anxiety, low self-esteem, or feelings of trauma, embracing a growth mindset can significantly impact their BJJ journey and overall personal development. In this subchapter, we will explore the key elements of a growth mindset and how they can be applied to the practice of BJJ.

A growth mindset encourages individuals to view challenges as opportunities for growth rather than obstacles to success. In the context of BJJ, this means embracing the struggles that come with learning new techniques or rolling with more experienced practitioners. For sedentary individuals or those who may have previously felt limited by their physical capabilities, recognizing that improvement is possible through consistent effort can foster resilience. This shift in perspective can transform feelings of frustration into motivation, helping practitioners push through their discomfort and ultimately build confidence in their abilities.

Another critical aspect of a growth mindset is the importance of feedback. In BJJ, constructive criticism from coaches and peers is invaluable for improvement. For those who may have experienced trauma or self-doubt, receiving feedback can be challenging. However, viewing feedback as a tool for growth rather than a personal attack can enhance emotional regulation and resilience. By integrating this mindset, practitioners can learn to appreciate the insights offered by others, allowing them to refine their skills and develop a more profound sense of self-worth.

Setting personal goals is an integral part of the growth mindset, particularly in the context of BJJ. Whether the goal is to achieve a new belt rank, master a specific technique, or improve overall fitness, having clear objectives can provide direction and purpose. For individuals seeking to overcome anxiety or build mental toughness, breaking larger goals into smaller, achievable steps can create a sense of accomplishment, reinforcing the belief that progress is attainable. This approach not only fosters a sense of achievement but also encourages continuous learning and adaptation, essential traits in both BJJ and life.

Finally, embracing a growth mindset can empower individuals, particularly women, to take charge of their BJJ journey and personal development. By fostering an environment that values growth, resilience, and emotional intelligence, practitioners can create supportive communities that uplift one another. This sense of camaraderie can be especially beneficial for those dealing with stress and trauma, as it provides a safe space for exploration and growth. Ultimately, understanding and adopting a growth mindset can transform the BJJ experience, turning it into a powerful tool for personal growth, emotional regulation, and self-empowerment.

Tools for Developing Resilience

Developing resilience is a multifaceted process that can be significantly enhanced through the practice of

Brazilian Jiu-Jitsu (BJJ). One of the primary tools for cultivating resilience is the structured environment of BJJ training. The consistent practice of techniques and sparring sessions fosters a sense of discipline and routine, which can be crucial for individuals seeking to manage anxiety and stress. In this setting, practitioners learn to confront challenges head-on, adapting to the dynamic nature of their opponents and the training environment. This adaptability is essential for resilience, as it prepares individuals to navigate life's unpredictability with greater confidence.

Another effective tool for developing resilience in BJJ is the supportive community that surrounds the sport. Training with others creates a sense of camaraderie and belonging, which can be particularly beneficial for individuals who may feel isolated due to their struggles with anxiety or low self-esteem. The encouragement from training partners and instructors can bolster confidence, allowing participants to push through their limits and celebrate their successes, no matter how small. This communal aspect reinforces the idea that resilience is not solely an individual endeavor; rather, it is often cultivated in the company of others who share similar goals and challenges.

Emotional intelligence plays a vital role in resilience, and BJJ offers a unique platform for enhancing this skill. As practitioners engage with their emotions during training—whether experiencing frustration, fear, or exhilaration—they learn to recognize and manage these feelings effectively. Instructors can integrate discussions about emotional responses and coping strategies into their coaching, helping students understand their emotional landscape. This awareness not only aids in personal growth but also equips practitioners with the tools needed to handle stress in other areas of their lives, ultimately contributing to greater mental toughness.

Goal setting is another powerful tool for resilience, and BJJ encourages this practice through its structured progression. Whether it's mastering a new technique, preparing for a competition, or achieving a personal milestone, setting specific, measurable goals can significantly enhance one's motivation and focus. This process teaches individuals the importance of perseverance and patience, as they learn that setbacks are often part of the journey. By recognizing that progress in BJJ mirrors life's challenges, practitioners can apply these lessons to other aspects of their lives, reinforcing their ability to overcome obstacles.

Lastly, BJJ serves as a means of empowerment, particularly for women and individuals who have experienced trauma. The self-defense skills learned in BJJ not only enhance physical safety but also instill a sense of confidence and agency. This empowerment is crucial for developing resilience, as it encourages individuals to take control of their narratives and confront their fears. Coupled with emotional regulation techniques learned during training, practitioners become equipped to handle stress and adversity more effectively. As they navigate their personal growth journeys, the tools gained through BJJ can lead to profound transformations, ultimately turning trauma into triumph.

The Role of BJJ in Cultivating a Resilient Mindset

The practice of Brazilian Jiu-Jitsu (BJJ) goes beyond physical self-defense; it serves as a powerful tool for cultivating a resilient mindset. For adults, especially those who may be experiencing anxiety or stress, engaging in BJJ provides an environment where challenges are not only faced but embraced. Each roll on the mat presents an opportunity to confront fears and uncertainties, transforming them into moments of growth. This process encourages practitioners to develop a mindset that views obstacles as opportunities rather than threats, fostering a sense of resilience that can be applied in various aspects of life.

As individuals engage in BJJ, they encounter both physical and mental challenges that require persistence and adaptability. Overcoming difficult training sessions, learning new techniques, and sparring with more experienced partners all contribute to building mental toughness. For those who have faced trauma, the practice of BJJ can be particularly transformative. It encourages individuals to confront their vulnerabilities in a safe environment, allowing for healing and personal growth. Each success on the mat, whether it be mastering a technique or winning a match, reinforces a sense of accomplishment and boosts self-esteem.

BJJ also plays a significant role in emotional regulation. The intense focus required during training helps practitioners cultivate mindfulness, allowing them to manage stress and anxiety more effectively. This is especially beneficial for sedentary individuals or those who may feel overwhelmed by life's pressures. The physical exertion involved in BJJ serves as a natural outlet for stress, while the community aspect fosters connections with others who share similar struggles. As practitioners learn to navigate their emotions on the mat, they develop essential emotional intelligence skills that translate to their daily lives.

For women, BJJ offers unique opportunities for empowerment and self-confidence. The sport promotes the idea that strength comes in many forms, encouraging female practitioners to embrace their capabilities and challenge societal norms. As women learn to defend themselves and engage in rigorous training, they cultivate a sense of agency and resilience that can significantly impact their personal and professional lives. This empowerment is crucial for women who have experienced trauma, as it fosters a renewed sense of self-worth and the ability to navigate challenges with courage.

Ultimately, the journey through Brazilian Jiu-Jitsu is a pathway to personal growth and goal setting. Practitioners learn to set realistic objectives, whether related to their technique, fitness levels, or competition goals. The process of striving for these goals, coupled with the inevitable setbacks, teaches valuable lessons about perseverance and resilience. As individuals progress in their BJJ journey, they not only become stronger martial artists but also more resilient individuals, equipped to face life's challenges with a newfound confidence and determination.

CHAPTER 10

Moving Forward: The Impact of BJJ on Life Beyond the Mat

Long-term Benefits of Practicing BJJ

Practicing Brazilian Jiu-Jitsu (BJJ) offers a multitude of long-term benefits that extend well beyond physical fitness. One of the most impactful advantages is the significant reduction in anxiety and stress levels. Engaging in BJJ requires intense focus and concentration, which naturally diverts attention from daily worries and stressors. During training, individuals find themselves in a flow state where they can forget about external pressures. This immersive experience not only fosters immediate relief from anxiety but also cultivates coping strategies that can be applied in everyday life, leading to a more resilient mindset over time.

BJJ serves as an excellent platform for building confidence and self-esteem. As practitioners progress through the ranks, they experience tangible improvements in their skills and technique. Each small victory on the mat, whether it's successfully executing a submission or defending against an opponent, contributes to a growing sense of self-efficacy. This newfound confidence often transcends the dojo, empowering individuals to tackle challenges in their personal and professional lives with a more assertive attitude. For many, this transformation is life-changing, enabling them to pursue goals they may have previously deemed unattainable.

Emotional intelligence is another crucial area enhanced by consistent BJJ practice. The sport teaches valuable lessons in empathy, patience, and communication as practitioners engage with partners of varying skill levels and backgrounds. Coaches and students alike learn to read non-verbal cues, adapt their strategies, and respond to the emotions of others in a constructive manner. This integration of emotional intelligence into BJJ not only improves interpersonal relationships but also plays a vital role in creating a supportive training environment. Over time, this development fosters a greater understanding of oneself and others, which is essential for personal and professional growth.

For individuals overcoming trauma, BJJ can be a powerful tool for building mental toughness. The challenges faced on the mat mirror those encountered in life, teaching practitioners to persevere in the face of adversity. The discipline required in training helps individuals develop resilience, enabling them to confront their fears and anxieties. As they learn to navigate difficult situations during sparring and competitions, they build the mental fortitude needed to deal with past trauma. This process can be profoundly therapeutic, facilitating healing and personal growth in a safe and supportive community.

BJJ promotes personal growth and goal setting in a unique way. The structured nature of belt progression and competition provides clear milestones for practitioners to strive towards. This goal-oriented approach encourages individuals to set both short-term and long-term objectives, fostering a sense of purpose and direction in their training. As they achieve these goals, practitioners experience a sense of accomplishment that motivates them to pursue new challenges, whether in BJJ or other areas of their lives. This continual cycle of setting and achieving goals not only reinforces self-discipline but also contributes to a deeper understanding of one's capabilities, paving the way for sustained personal development.

Building a Lifestyle of Resilience

Building a lifestyle of resilience is essential for individuals navigating the complexities of modern life, especially for those who have faced trauma or mental health challenges. Brazilian Jiu-Jitsu (BJJ) offers a unique framework that fosters resilience through physical and mental engagement. Practicing BJJ encourages individuals to confront their fears, develop coping mechanisms, and build a strong sense of self-efficacy. This martial art teaches practitioners how to face adversity on the mat, translating these lessons into everyday life. The journey of resilience begins with recognizing that setbacks are a part of growth, and BJJ provides the perfect environment to practice this principle.

One of the key elements in building resilience through BJJ is the emphasis on problem-solving. Each roll on the mat presents new challenges that require quick thinking and adaptability. As practitioners grapple with opponents, they learn to assess situations, anticipate moves, and develop strategies to overcome obstacles. This mental engagement enhances cognitive flexibility, allowing individuals to approach life's challenges with a more constructive mindset. Over time, this problem-solving mindset cultivates not only resilience but also confidence, as individuals realize their ability to navigate difficulties effectively.

Emotional regulation is another vital component of resilience, and BJJ serves as an excellent medium for developing this skill. During training, athletes are pushed physically and emotionally, often encountering frustration, fatigue, and even fear. Learning to manage these emotions in a high-pressure environment fosters greater emotional intelligence. Practitioners become adept at recognizing and controlling their emotional responses, enabling them to handle stress and anxiety in their daily lives. This emotional regulation is particularly beneficial for those who have experienced trauma, as it equips them with tools to cope with triggers and build a more stable emotional foundation.

Building a lifestyle of resilience through BJJ also encourages a sense of community and support. The camaraderie found in BJJ schools creates a safe space for individuals to share their experiences, challenges, and triumphs. This supportive environment fosters connections that can be incredibly healing, especially for those dealing with feelings of isolation or low self-esteem. Practitioners not only learn from their instructors but also from each other, reinforcing the idea that they are not alone in their struggles. The bonds formed within the BJJ community can significantly enhance personal growth and resilience, providing motivation and encouragement during difficult times.

Integrating BJJ into a lifestyle of resilience requires setting realistic goals and celebrating progress, no matter how small. Goal setting is a powerful tool for personal development, and BJJ provides a clear pathway for this practice. From earning new belts to mastering techniques, each achievement reinforces the notion that perseverance leads to success. Setting and achieving these goals instills a sense of accomplishment, further strengthening resilience. For those who may feel overwhelmed by the demands of life, BJJ offers a structured approach to personal growth, empowering individuals to transform their challenges into triumphs.

Inspiring Others through Personal Transformation

Inspiring others through personal transformation is a powerful concept that resonates deeply within the Brazilian Jiu-Jitsu community. Many individuals come to BJJ seeking not only physical improvement but also a means to navigate their emotional and psychological struggles. The journey of mastering this martial art often reflects a broader metamorphosis, where practitioners learn to confront and overcome their fears, insecurities, and past traumas. As they evolve on the mats, they become living testimonies of resilience, illustrating how dedication and perseverance can lead to profound changes in one's life.

The process of transformation in Brazilian Jiu-Jitsu involves much more than technical skills; it encompasses the development of mental toughness and emotional intelligence. As practitioners face opponents who challenge their strength, agility, and strategy, they also confront their internal barriers. This confrontation fosters a unique environment for growth, where individuals learn to manage anxiety and stress, thereby finding relief through physical exertion and mental focus. By sharing their experiences, those who have transformed their lives through BJJ can inspire newcomers, showing them that they too can achieve their goals and improve their well-being.

Building confidence and self-esteem is a significant outcome of engaging with Brazilian Jiu-Jitsu. Many participants, especially those who may have felt marginalized or insecure in their lives, discover a sense of empowerment on the mat. Each success, whether it's mastering a new technique or overcoming a challenging opponent, serves as a building block for self-worth. As these individuals share their stories of triumph, they encourage others, particularly those who are overweight or sedentary, to step outside their comfort zones. This ripple effect not only transforms individuals but can also reshape communities, fostering a culture of support and encouragement.

Integrating emotional intelligence into BJJ coaching enhances the potential for transformation. Coaches who understand the emotional and psychological aspects of their students' journeys can tailor their approaches to meet individual needs. By fostering an atmosphere of empathy and understanding, these coaches help students navigate their emotional landscapes, providing tools for emotional regulation and resilience. This supportive environment cultivates not only skilled practitioners but also individuals who are adept at managing their emotions, thereby inspiring others to embark on their personal growth journeys.

Finally, Brazilian Jiu-Jitsu serves as a powerful tool for female empowerment, particularly in a world that often challenges women's confidence and emotional expression. Female practitioners often find strength in the community and the practice itself, which encourages assertiveness and resilience. As women share their transformative experiences, they inspire others, creating a network of support that promotes personal growth and goal setting. In this way, BJJ becomes a platform for women to reclaim their narratives, foster emotional regulation, and inspire others to pursue their own paths of transformation.

About the Author

JOAO CRUS was born in Brasilia, Brazil, and moved to Rio de Janeiro when he was 17 years old. In his youth, he was very active and athletic in swimming. He started his initial Martial Arts training with Karate at the age of 22 and earned the rank of brown belt. Just before he was about to test for his black belt, he stumbled upon Brazilian Jiu-Jitsu, and began secretly attending classes while he was still training Karate.

In his competitions in Karate, Joao won 5 State Tournaments and was 2nd place in a National Tournament in Rio de Janeiro, Brazil. However, once Joao had a taste of BJJ he no longer had the desire to complete his black belt in Karate, and began training BJJ full time in 1998.

Before he came to the United States, he earned his blue belt under Leonardo Castello Branco in Rio. In addition to his martial arts training, Joao was a strong competitor in WindSurfing and Sailing in Brazil. He won the amateur circuit 3 times in the Caribbean competitions.

Joao was a part of the sports and nutrition world as a top sales representative for Optimum Nutrition and started his own store in 1999. During this time, he developed a friendship with world renowned Carlson Gracie. Carlson would visit his store regularly, just to visit and talk about life. Years later when Joao began training in jiu-jitsu again, he became an instructor under Carlson Gracie.

Joao has been teaching Brazilian Jiu-Jitsu in the Austin area for two decades, and has operated his own school in Dripping Springs for sixteen years. A few years ago he expanded to Austin, and now owns and operates two jiu-jitsu schools in the Austin area.

Joao is considered to be an expert in teaching children jiu-jitsu, and many of the top Brazilian jiu-jitsu coaches and school owners have turned to him for advice on starting their own children's programs. He wrote a book called " Grapple with Emotions", about how Brazilian Jiu-Jitsu can be a tool to help children to become emotionally regulated. He has created numerous DVDs and video resources for instructors on teaching Brazilian jiu-jitsu, and has schools affiliated with him across the country and overseas. Joao speaks three languages, and has also traveled throughout Europe teaching seminars and spreading the art of Brazilian jiu-jitsu. He currently resides in Austin, TX, and when he's not teaching BJJ he enjoys outdoor activities such as rock climbing, hiking, tango dancing and swimming.